7

un you cecewots
and good humor.
Each teon menbe-
has a page —

Unsolicited *Molly*

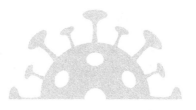

Unsolicited

96 Saws and Quips
from the
Wake of the Pandemic

Molly O'Dell

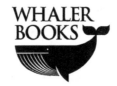

WHALER
BOOKS

1 3 5 7 9 10 8 6 4 2

Library of Congress Control Number: 2021914449

Unsolicited: 96 Saws and Quips from the Wake of the Pandemic
By Molly O'Dell
p. cm.

1. Reference—Quotations
2. Medical—Infectious Diseases
3. Self-Help—General

I. O'Dell, Molly 1954– II. Title.
ISBN 13: 978-1-7349136-6-8 (softcover : alk. paper)

Design by Karen Bowen

Whaler Books
An imprint of Mariner Media, Inc.
131 West 21st Street, Buena Vista, VA 24416
Tel: 540-264-0021 ▪ www.marinermedia.com

Printed in the United States of America

This book is printed on acid-free paper meeting the requirements of the American Standard for Permanence of Paper for Printed Library Materials.

Acknowledgments

Common understanding of the complex practice of public health has grown over the past year, and I am so privileged to have learned from and worked with some of the best professionals in the field during my years of service for the Virginia Department of Health, starting with Reba Weeks, Glenna Sprinkle, Helen Morris, and Nancy Welch in 1983.

Responding to the pandemic of 2020 was an unprecedented public health challenge, which shed light on the work carried out by local and regional citizens. It is impossible to name each individual, but I am forever grateful for the efforts of every single health department employee and volunteer from the Alleghany and Roanoke City Health Districts and Southwest Virginia, the reporters who covered our work and promoted our recommendations, and the scientists and staff at the Fralin Biomedical Research Institute who developed our region's COVID testing capacity.

Thanks are also due to Sue Cantrell, Duncan Adams, and Hope White for improving this manuscript and Karen Bowen who helped the manuscript become a token of transformation for all of us who lived through the pandemic and for those who diligently worked to mitigate the effect of SARS CoV-2 in our communities.

Preface

What's important during a pandemic turns out to be important, period.

On Saint Patrick's Day, 2020, I left retirement and returned to the Virginia Department of Health to lead the epidemiologic response to SARS CoV-2 for the Alleghany and Roanoke City Health Districts in southwest Virginia. On that day the epidemiology team was a person of one. And the emergency response system was also a person of one.

Within several days, we managed to construct an incident command structure and an epidemiologic response team (epi team) and to develop protocols to assure the health and safety of our employees, patients, partners, and citizens. Our first epi team meeting commenced March 19, the day of our first confirmed COVID-19 case report. We continued to meet for two hundred and ninety-one days.

Our epi team was composed of three epidemiologists, an infectious disease physician, an environmental health specialist, a public health nurse supervisor, five public health nurses, a public health physician, and me. We lived our lives individually, but we spent most of our waking hours problem-solving and communicating with one another as we learned everything on the fly. We used part of our team meeting time, every day, to verify our interpretation of new information and guidance, so we communicated a unified message to all people and organizations in our community. We also processed what we encountered during our previous day's work.

It was impossible to ignore the various ways human beings responded to recommended changes in individual and community life as the days rolled on. Members of our team got married, became sick, planted gardens, lost loved ones, changed jobs, birthed lambs, and harvested vegetables. Everyone was encouraged to practice self-care, take time off, and identify and train a back-up. The intensity of the work was tremendous and all of us worked around the clock when necessary. It was not uncommon for me to talk with the regional jail superintendent as I changed into my pajamas at ten thirty at night. We shared these absurdities with our teammates whenever possible.

The recognition of the role of public health and epidemiology in the lives of all citizens has never been greater. This past year has exposed the best and worst of local, state, and national public health systems. As humans working this pandemic, we were as successful as our systems allowed. Our systems were decades behind and became politically influenced.

Balancing individual rights with the assurance of community health has never been trickier.

The saws and quips on these pages presented themselves during our incident command meetings and the epi team's two-hundred-and-ninety-one days of work together. These saws and quips flashed from my journal one weekend as I pondered what I was supposed to have learned from all those hours working to impede the spread of SARS CoV-2.

As epidemiologists and public health workers, we sure worked hard. We also mined humor and learned all there was to know about SARS CoV-2 and about our species, homo sapiens. And then, as new science and behaviors emerged, we relearned it all over again.

A contact of
a contact is
not a contact.

"Never turn down help
unless you are eating."

–Amy Stinnett White

Pay attention to
your dreams.

If you hear or read
a word or term you
don't know, look it up.

Once someone you love turns eighteen, stop offering unsolicited advice.

"Being approximately right most of the time is better than being precisely right occasionally."

—*Anonymous*

Learning is not
optional during
a pandemic.

Being prepared
is the best way to
initiate a response
to any challenge.

Keep a comprehensive
rolodex on your phone,
in your computer, or
on note cards.

In the middle
of a pandemic
or magnificent
celebration, the
execution of
menial tasks is
still required.

Understand the clade*
you are dealing with.

*A clade is a group of biological species that
include all descendants of one common
ancestor.

Trim the wick
before lighting
a candle.

Pay attention to
the questions of
reporters. They
know what people
are asking.

This virus is
behaving exactly
like it's supposed
to; human
beings are not.

"Follow the grain of
your own wood."

–*Howard Thurman*

Infection control
in nursing homes
is an oxymoron.

Life is a lot easier
if you live below
your means.

How our systems
support the least
among us is how
we should grade
our systems.

When a peaceful-looking lion appears in your dream, take encouragement and feel strong. You are headed in the right direction.

Cultivate variety in
all aspects of life;
differences make the
best conversations,
and sameness
creates empathy.

Always return
phone calls by
the end of the
day, even on the
weekend during
lambing season.

Subscribe to
your local
newspaper.

"Profanity offers
spiritual relief
unavailable
through prayer."

—*Anthony de Mello*

Show respect to
meat packers,
farmers, grocers,
and those who work
in manufacturing;
our daily lives
depend on them.

Sometimes we
must choose
between being
right and being
in a relationship.

It's never the
wrong choice
to be polite.

"Indeed" utters
affirmation
and collegiality
during an intense
conversation.

It's best to let public health professionals handle public health matters.

Zoom, click,
call, mute is
not music.

When it comes to
bobby pins, you get
what you pay for.

One COVID year
equals the amount
of new information
assimilated and put into
practice in one day.

"When barraged with tragedy, loss, and hopelessness day after day, practice four things: laugh, think, cry, and never lose sight of where we started, where we are at, and where we want to be. These things keep us grounded and level."

–Tim Knight, Lt.
Virginia State Police

Pay attention to
expiration dates.

If Michael
Friedlander says
he'll have PCR
testing available
in six months,
believe him.

Share good
news widely.

When you're about
to give a live TV
simulcast and all
you can think about
is a synonym for
reagent, make sure
you are getting
enough sleep.

There is no
such thing as a
quick question.

Always have
someone edit your
written work.

There is no way to accurately predict the slope of an epi curve.

If you can't honor
a commitment
to a meeting or
social engagement,
let the organizer
know, preferably
ahead of time.

Buy estate jewelry;
there are plenty of
gorgeous stones
and precious metals
available without
digging up more.

"Can you hear me?" is not a sentence.

(This one's for the governor.)

It's not good for
morale to change the
state performance
planning and
evaluation system
in the middle of a
pandemic.

Don't make work
for other people.

Avoid admission
to jail during a
pandemic.

When you receive
a phone call from a
stranger, adopt an
attitude of curiosity.
Your next best
friend could be the
superintendent of
the regional jail.

Trust the people who answer the phones. They have nothing to lose and deserve your support.

When you dream
you are weeding
the pachysandra
and the furry noses
of a chocolate lab
and possum with a
hairless tail appear,
consider taking a
vacation.

"Even when we
learn quite a
bit, it doesn't
mean we know
anything."

—Tom Kerkering

During an infectious disease outbreak, remember that your actions will either promote the spread of the disease or prevent it.

Recognize others
always and yourself
as little as possible.

Believe me, there
is a world of
difference between
a for-profit and a
not-for-profit health
system.

Good people
work in less than
good systems.

You can always rely
on medical students.

If you dream about someone being disgusted with you, consider who you are disgusted with!

Experiential
learning is messy.

Numbers are
important,
trends more so.

Never underestimate the power of a close-knit community!

Having a positive
COVID test makes
some people feel
important.

How we handle
our trash is just
as important as
how we handle
our food.

Integrity is
seeing a pair
of cottontails
hop down
Rabbit Run.

To reduce feedback
in a virtual meeting,
simply mute your
phone or audio when
you're not speaking.

Some people are at
their best telling lies.

Practice helping others know and practice what they do best.

Females are usually
the medical leaders
in a household.

When you dream about a panda bear, examine how balanced or off-balanced your life has become.

Never lose sight of
what's happening
on the margins.

Some school board members aren't from here, don't have children, and are simply political animals.

Never underestimate
the ignorance of the
wealthy and well-
educated.

Relationships
wax and wane
throughout life, so
avoid severing any
of them.

When solving a
problem or making a
diagnosis, there's no
substitute for seeing
the situation with
your own two eyes.

If you dream
about monkeys,
it's time to play
more with family
and friends.

Actions, not
words, reveal
the true
character of
a person.

When you dream
about wildebeest,
consider what's
overwhelming you,
what needs changing,
and assess your
family ties.

Keep any fossil
you find. They
are precious.

Learning in school
is actually more
important than
playing sports.

"We hang in the
balance of the past
and the possible."

–Thomas Merton

Be wary of people
who don't know what
they don't know or
can't own what they
don't know.

Support funding
for public health at
the local, state, and
national level.

Clinicians, if you order a lab test, x-ray, or study, it's your responsibility to check for the results and share the results with the patient as soon as they are available.

Don't ask anyone
to do something
you have not
already done or
aren't willing to
do yourself.

When people are sick or tired or hungry or stressed, give them lots of slack and forgiveness.

Tell the truth.
Don't cheat or lie.

Unions still provide an important form of accountability. Just ask me about one of our railroad companies.

Always check the
source document
before quoting data.

Multi-layered well-fitted face coverings are better than single layer gators for preventing the spread of SARS CoV-2 to and from the wearer.

Trust each person you
meet until they give
you a reason not to.

The longer you are
close to another person
the greater the chance
you will learn or catch
something from that
other person.

Don't squander
your quarantine.

Recovery is a
loaded word.

For the next several
years, avoid using
the words pivot,
spike protein,
surge, or zoom.

It never works
to compare your
insides to somebody
else's outsides.

Be kind; it's always appreciated.

Get vaccinated; it's
a responsibility of
being a good citizen.

Try to be a good neighbor.

If you dream of a
person disrobing in
public, it's likely your
subconscious rejecting
the sequestration of
shock you experience
at what people do,
where they do it, when
and why they do it, and
who they do it to.

About the Author

Molly O'Dell was born and raised in southwest Virginia, where she spent thirty of her professional life years practicing medicine and public health. She graduated from Longwood College in 1976, the Medical College of Virginia in 1980, and received an MFA in poetry from the University of Nebraska in 2009. A month after her second book, *Care is A Four-Letter Verb,* was accepted for publication by WordTech Editions, she left retirement to lead the pandemic response at home and is now grateful to read, write, hike, dig in the dirt, and float Virginia waterways as much as each day allows. To learn more, visit www.doctormolly.net.